T0193083

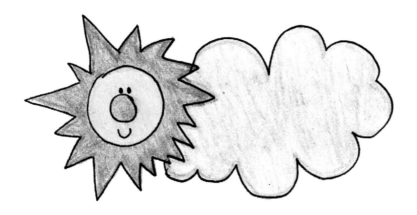
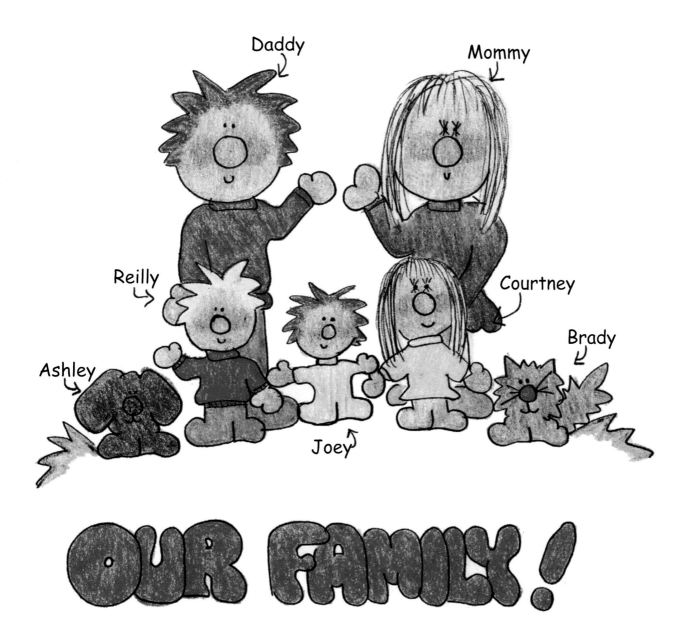

Order this book online at www.trafford.com
or email orders@trafford.com

Most Trafford titles are also available at major online book retailers.

Trafford PUBLISHING® www.trafford.com

North America & international
toll-free: 844 688 6899 (USA & Canada)
fax: 812 355 4082

Our mission is to efficiently provide the world's finest, most comprehensive book publishing service, enabling every author to experience success. To find out how to publish your book, your way, and have it available worldwide, visit us online at www.trafford.com

DEDICATION

To my family including, my husband Ron, my children and their spouses - Wesley (Gail) Greer, Warren Greer, Lana Greer-Connell (Shaun) and my grandchildren Courtney, Reilly, Joey, and Natalie, and my Mom, Margaret McDonald.

ACKNOWLEDGMENTS

Dr Warren Hollis and Dr Elaine Chagnon for inspiring me to write this book. Louise Freeman for her help and friendship. My teacher Dr Anton Jayasuriya for his wisdom. Don Kealey for his encouragement and reading my book. Thanks to Marie Tysick for her suggestions. Stephen Bird for proofreading. Ivan and Elizabeth Bird for their constant support. Jan Buckland for the layout of the book. Larry Edmonds for his wonderful idea of using crayons for the drawings. Lenora Dowdall and Gail Dowdall for their kindness. To the following young readers who previewed this book and provided their valuable opinions; Seneid Burson, Ciaran Burson, Sarah Salisbury, Isis Bennet, Sage blacklavender, Adam Livingstone. Finally, my daughter-in-law, Gail Greer for her wonderful illustrations.

ISBN: 978-1-4120-1810-4 (sc)

Print information available on the last page.

Trafford rev. 02/07/2022

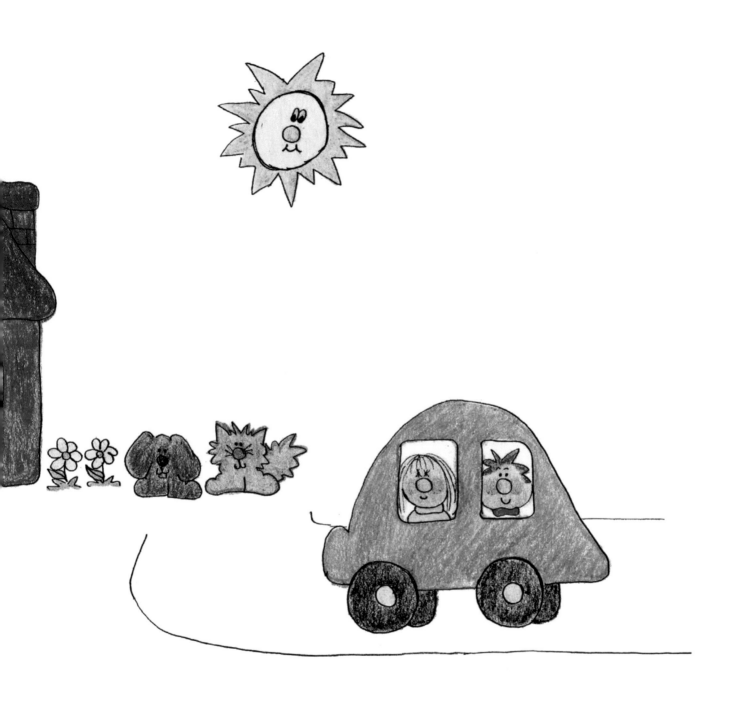

OUR FAMILY HAS AN APPOINTMENT TODAY
WITH THE ACUPUNCTURIST.

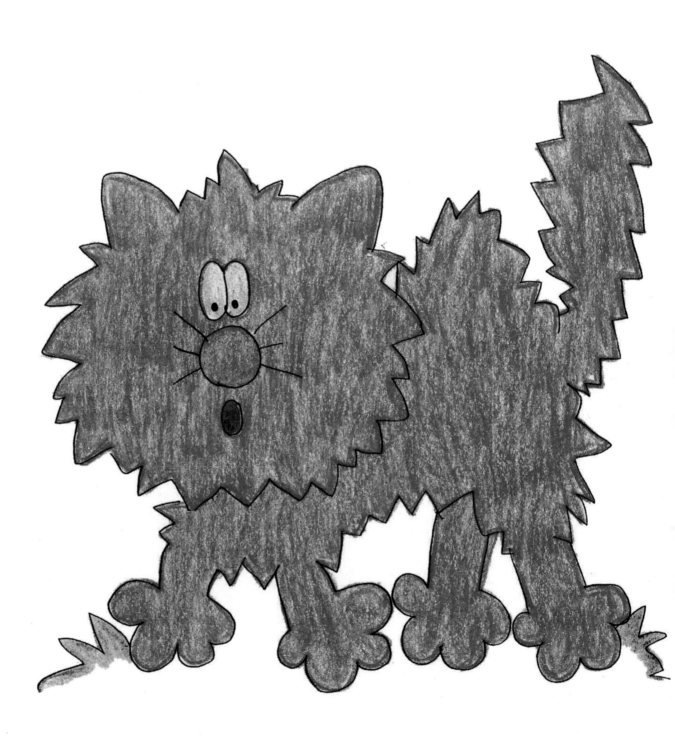

ARE WE GOING TOO?

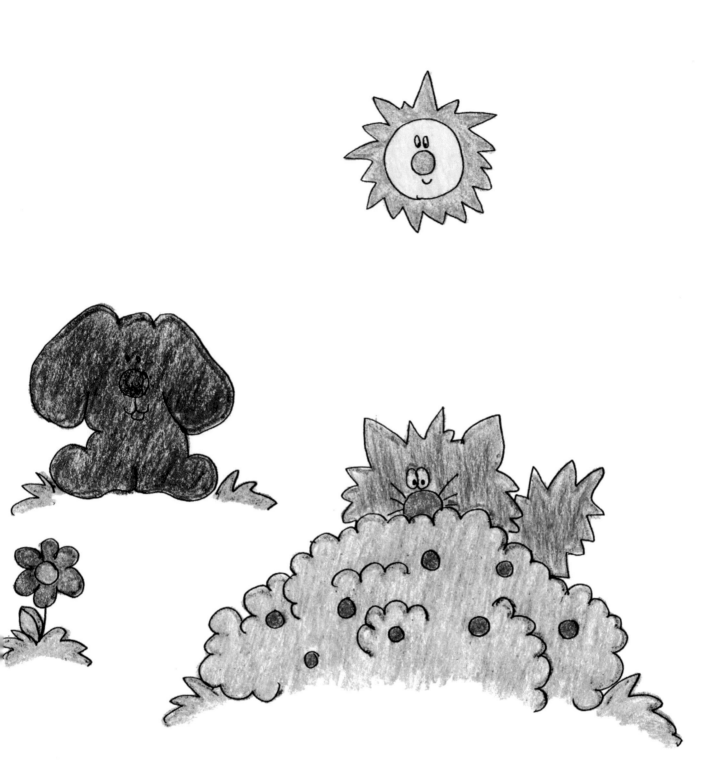

NO, NOT THIS TIME, BUT ACUPUNCTURE IS PRACTICALLY PAINLESS.

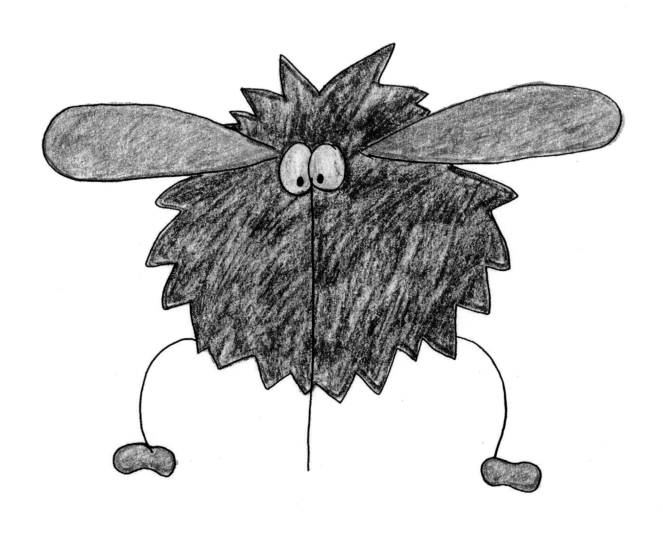

A MOSQUITO BITE IS FELT MORE THAN A VERY FINE
ACUPUNCTURE NEEDLE. THEY ARE PAPER THIN.

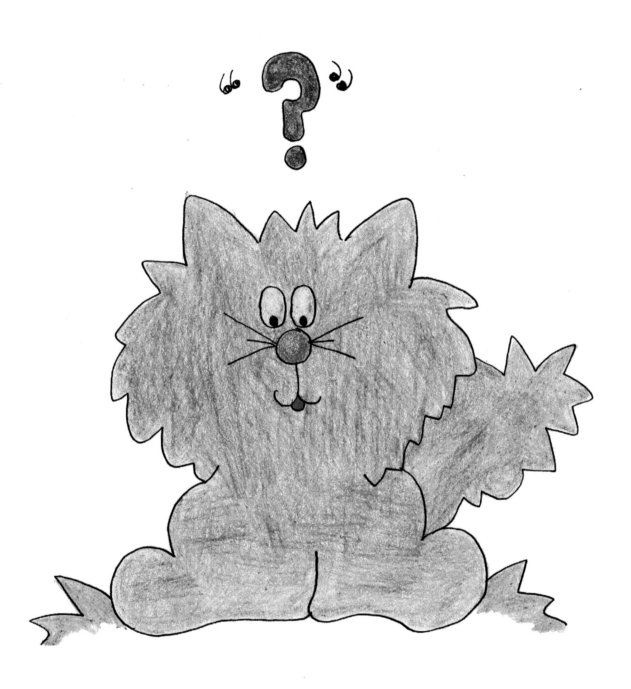

WHAT DOES ACUPUNCTURE MEAN?

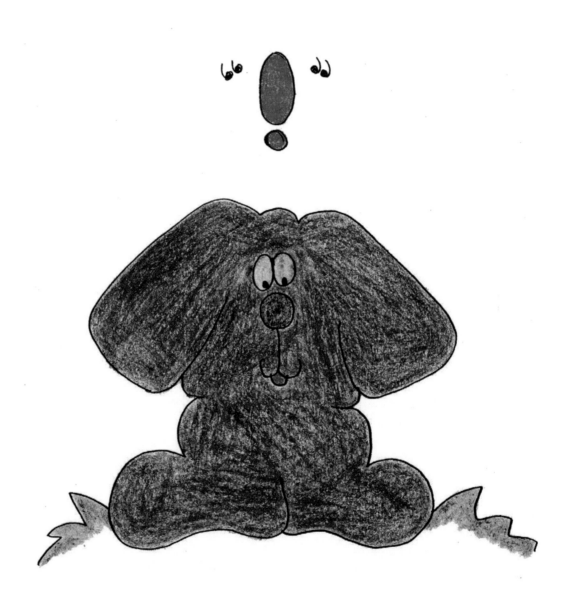

ACU IS THE LATIN WORD FOR NEEDLE, PUNCTURA IS THE LATIN WORD MEANING TO PUNCTURE. ACUPUNCTURE IS THE OLDEST MEDICAL STUDY IN THE WORLD. IT ORIGINATED OVER 5000 YEARS AGO.

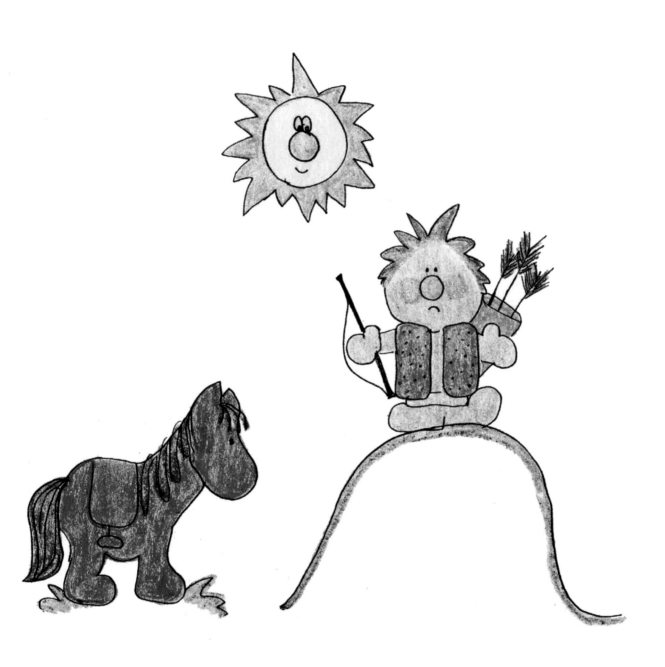

THERE ARE MANY THEORIES AS TO HOW ACUPUNCTURE BEGAN.

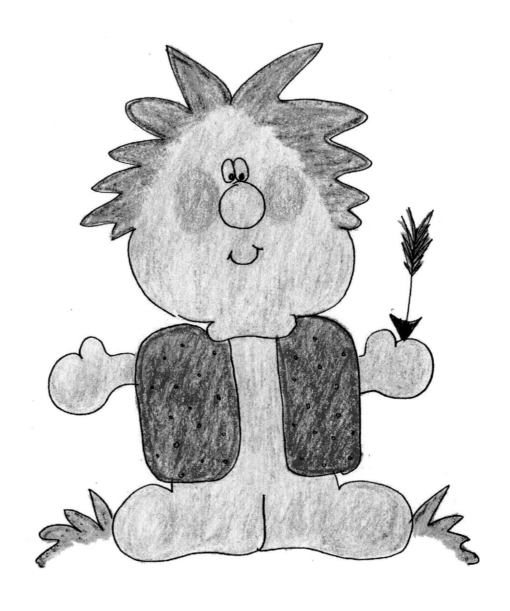

ONE IS THE STORY OF A WARRIOR WOUNDED BY AN ARROW.
WHEN THE ARROW WAS REMOVED, A DISEASE IN ANOTHER
PART OF HIS BODY BECAME WELL.

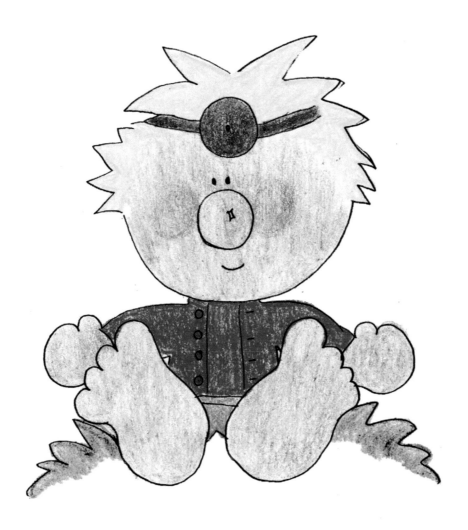

HAVE YOU EVER HEARD OF BARE-FOOT DOCTORS?
THIS NAME REFERS TO ACUPUNCTURISTS TRAINED TO
PROVIDE MEDICAL SERVICES IN RURAL CHINA.

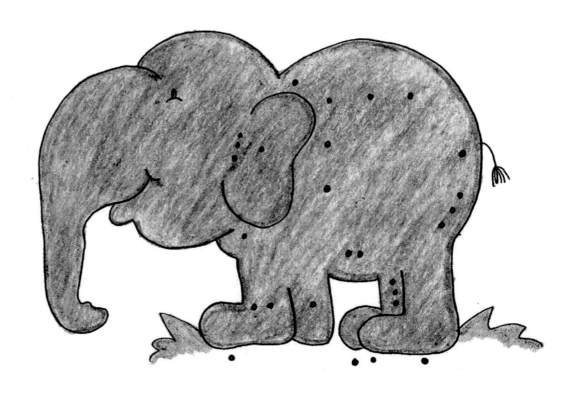

DID YOU KNOW THAT THE ASIAN ELEPHANT HAS
89 ACU (OR ACUPUNCTURE) POINTS? ELEPHANTS HAVE
ACUPUNCTURE WHEN THEY ARE SICK, OR TO ASSIST THEM
WHEN THEY CARRY HEAVY LOADS.

12

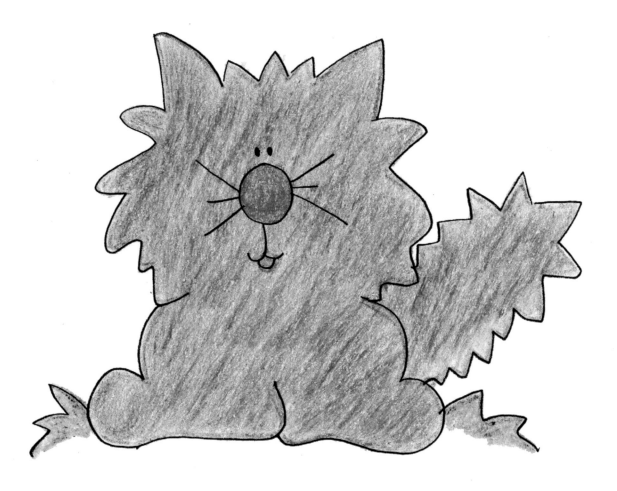

WHY IS OUR FAMILY VISITING THE ACUPUNCTURIST?

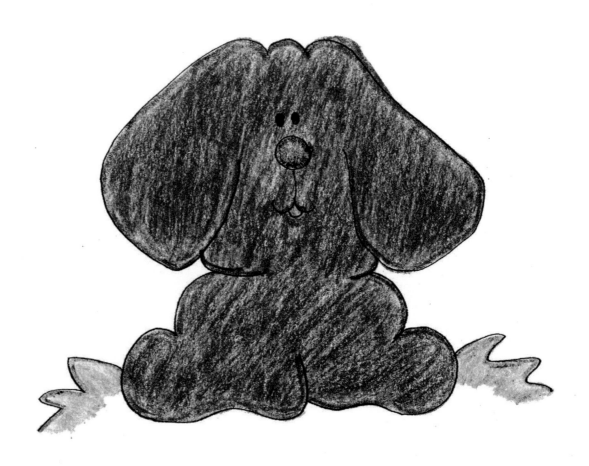

THEY ARE GOING FOR THEIR ONCE A YEAR CHECK-UP,
JUST AS THEY WOULD VISIT THEIR FAMILY DOCTOR.
ACUPUNCTURE HELPS KEEP YOUR WHOLE BODY HEALTHY.

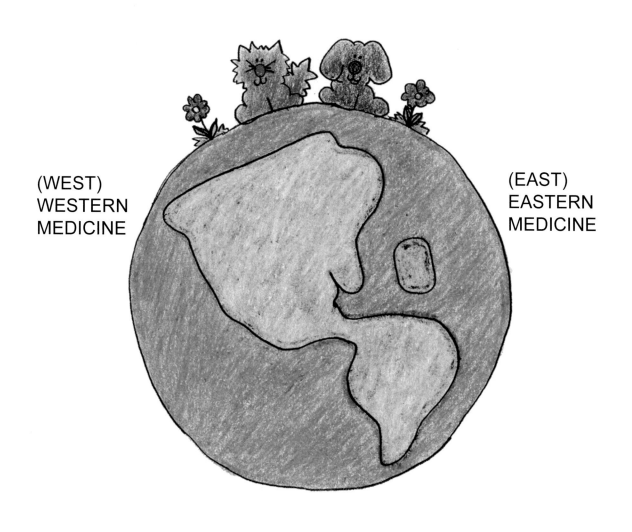

(WEST)
WESTERN
MEDICINE

(EAST)
EASTERN
MEDICINE

THE FAMILY DOCTOR IS REFERRED TO AS "WESTERN MEDICINE"
(FROM THE WEST), AND ACUPUNCTURE IS "CHINESE MEDICINE"
(FROM THE EAST).

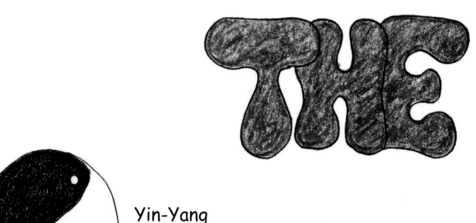

THE

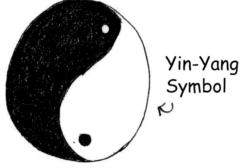

Yin-Yang
Symbol

Acupuncturist

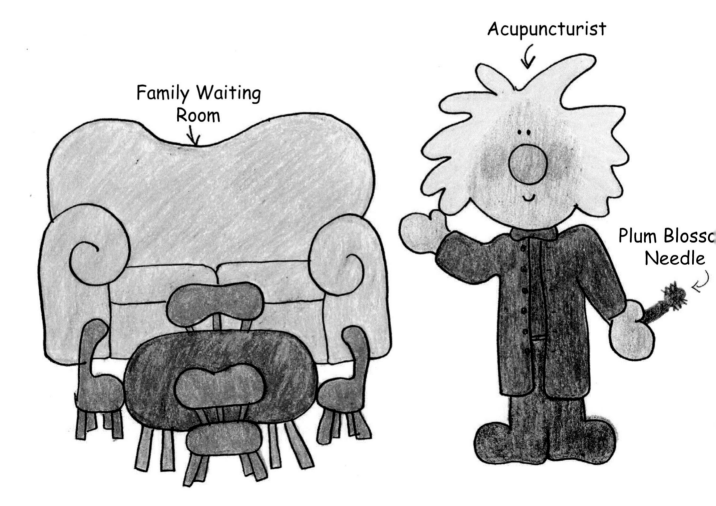

Family Waiting
Room

Plum Blosso
Needle

16

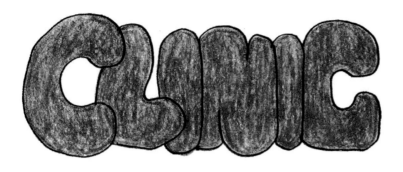

CLINIC

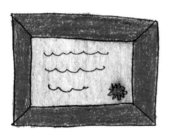
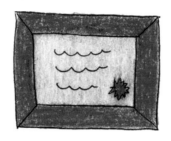

Desk

Acupuncture Table

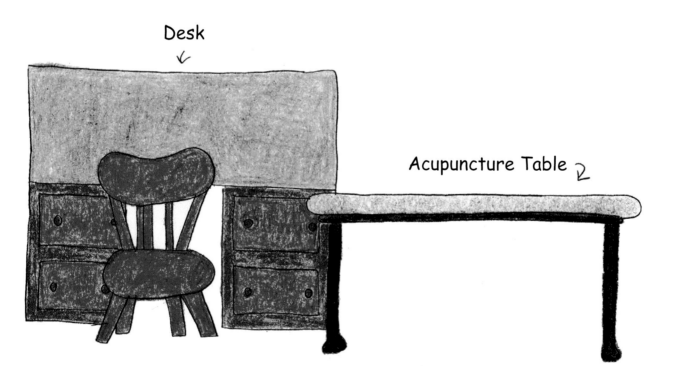

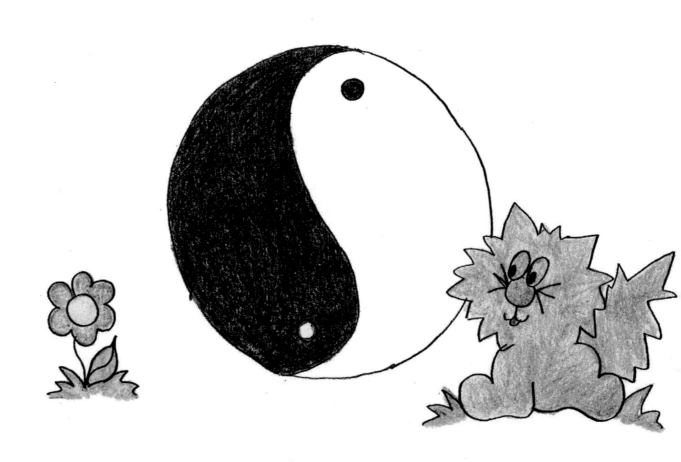

WHAT DOES THE CIRCLE WITH THE CURVED LINE MEAN?

18

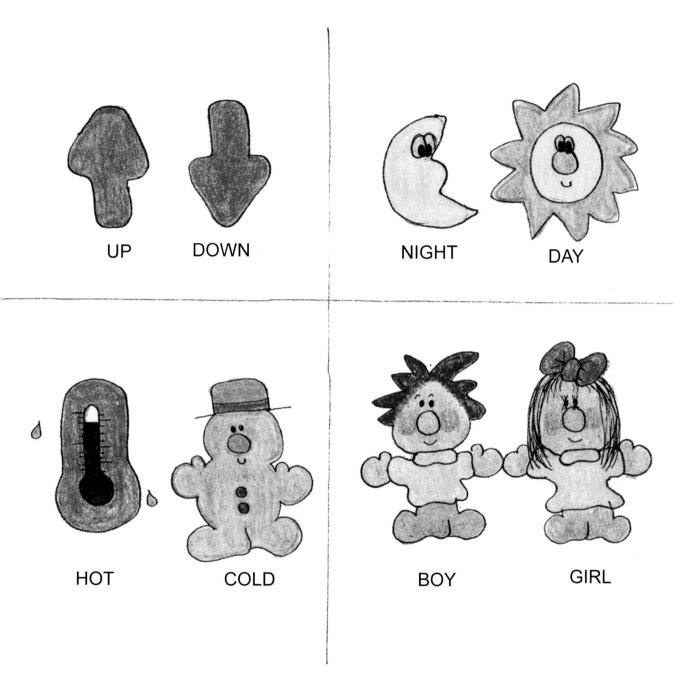

UP   DOWN

NIGHT   DAY

HOT   COLD

BOY   GIRL

IT IS CALLED YIN AND YANG. YIN AND YANG REPRESENTS
OUR BODY IN PERFECT BALANCE.

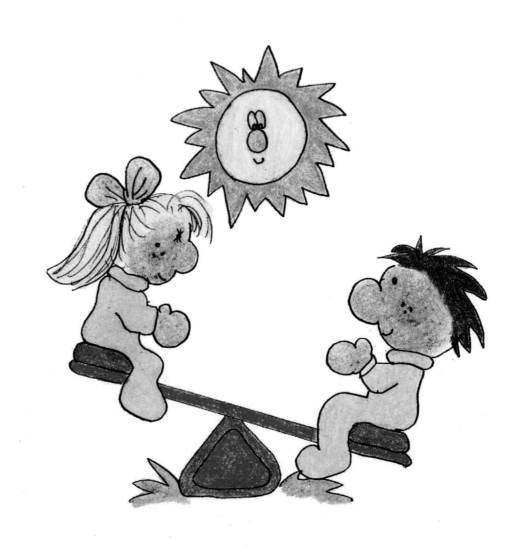

A TEETER TOTTER IS A GOOD EXAMPLE OF THE
OPPOSITES UP AND DOWN (YIN AND YANG).

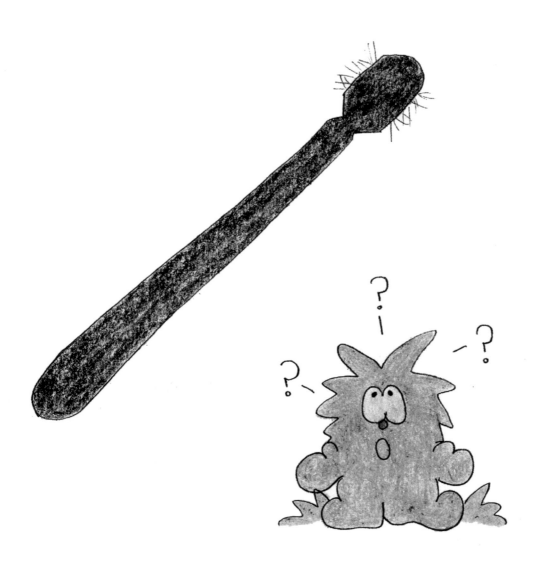

THE PLUM BLOSSOM NEEDLE IS VERY USEFUL IN TREATING
YOUNG CHILDREN AS WELL AS THE ELDERLY.

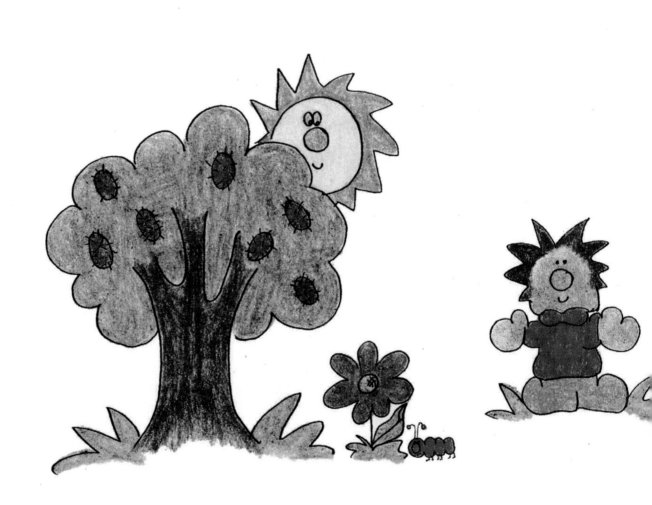

THESE NEEDLES ARE SIMILAR TO THE ONES ON THE
PLUM BLOSSOMS FROM THE PLUM BLOSSOM TREE.

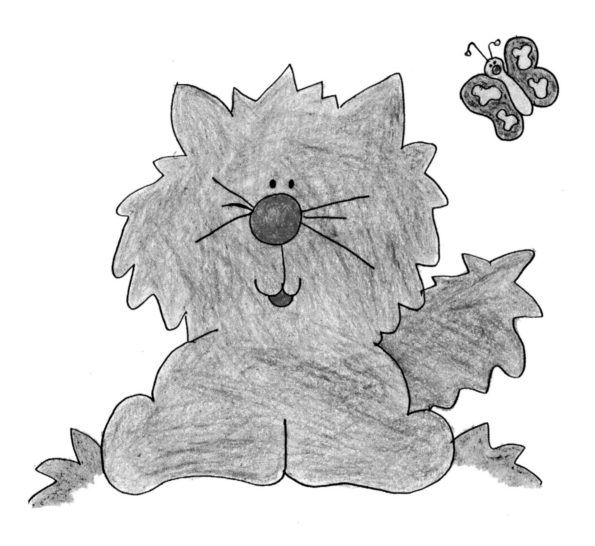

IF SOMEONE IS SICK, HOW DOES ACUPUNCTURE
MAKE THEM BETTER?

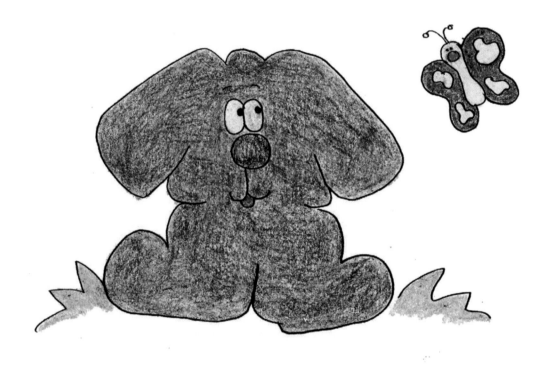

IN TRADITIONAL CHINESE MEDICINE, NETWORKS OF ENERGY CALLED "QI" (PRONOUNCED CHEE) FLOW THROUGH THE BODY ALONG NATURAL PATHWAYS (ALSO CALLED CHANNELS OR MERIDIANS). THESE PATHWAYS ARE INVISIBLE AREAS (YOU CANNOT SEE THEM). THE CHINESE BELIEVE THAT DISEASE GROWS WHEN THAT ENERGY IS BLOCKED. BY INSERTING VERY FINE NEEDLES AT PRECISE POSITIONS ALONG THESE PATHWAYS, THE BODY'S FLOW OF ENERGY IS RESTORED ALLOWING IT TO BALANCE AND BECOME WELL.

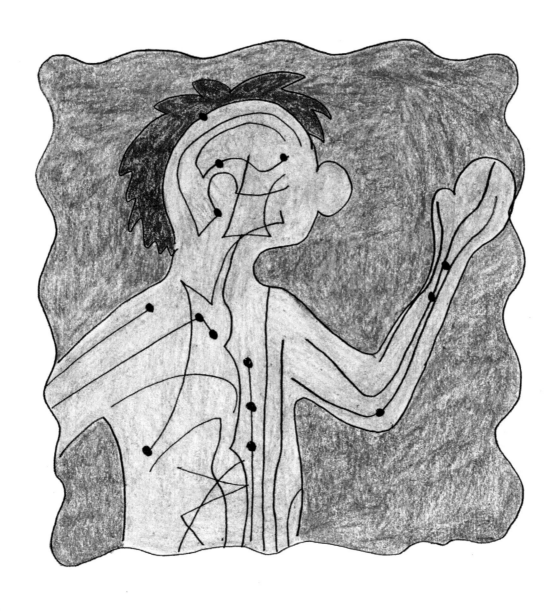

THERE ARE 12 PAIRED CHANNELS (PATHWAYS OR MERIDIANS)
AND 8 EXTRA CHANNELS ON OUR BODY AND, APPROXIMATELY
365 ACU (ACUPUNCTURE) POINTS.

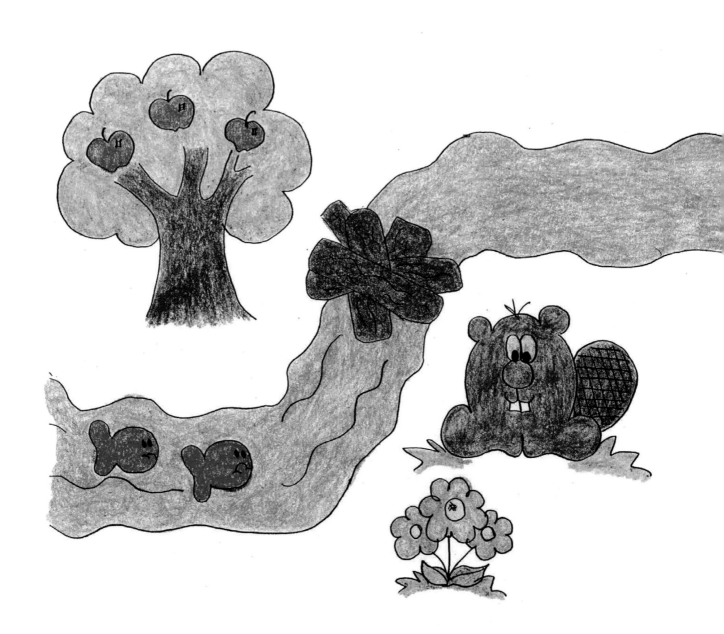

ANOTHER WAY TO EXPLAIN THE ENERGY FLOW IS TO COMPARE IT TO A FREE FLOWING RIVER. LET'S SAY A BEAVER MOVES IN AND DAMS THE RIVER WITH WOOD. THE FLOW OF THE WATER IS THEN BLOCKED.

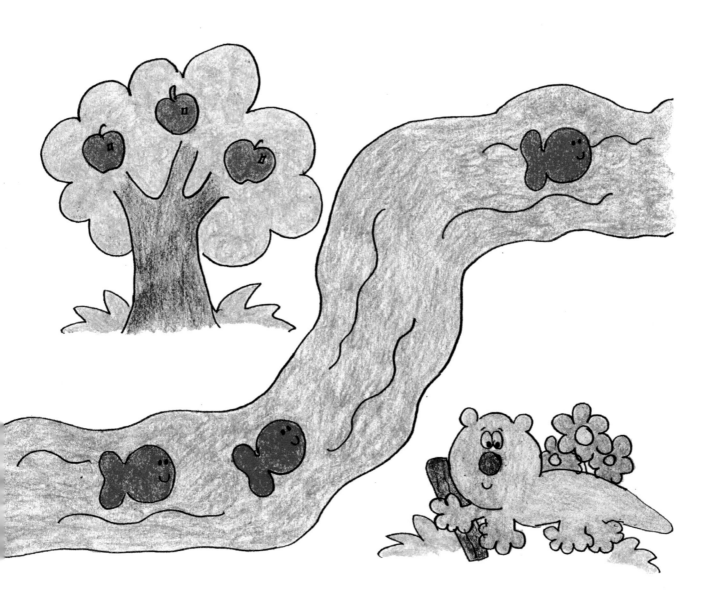

NOW LET'S PRETEND AN OTTER REMOVES THE WOOD
DESTROYING THE DAM. THE WATER IS THEN ABLE TO FLOW
FREELY JUST AS THE ENERGY FLOWS FREELY IN A HEALTHY BODY
- NOT TOO FAST AND NOT TOO SLOW.

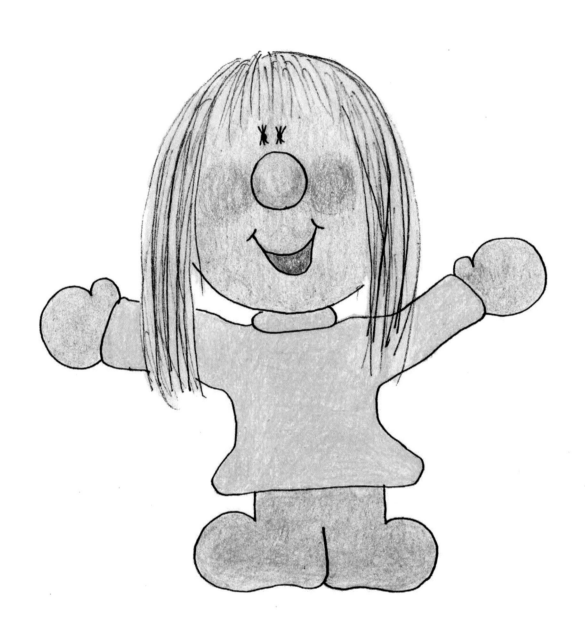

WE'RE BACK!

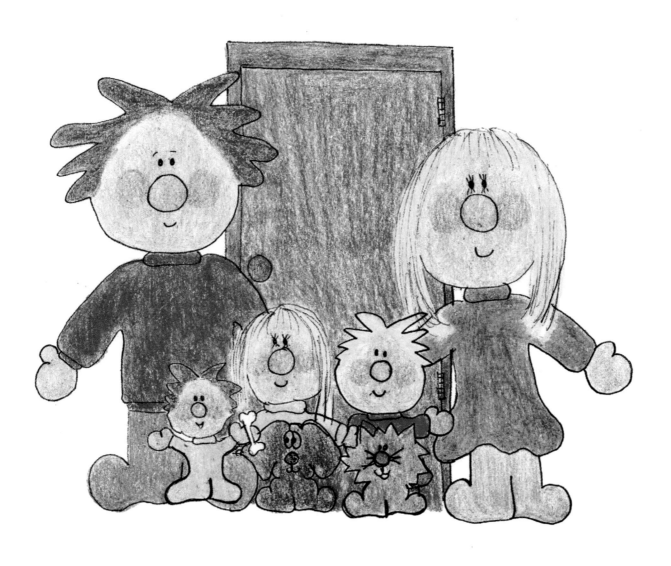

LOOK, OUR FAMILY IS BACK FROM THE ACUPUNCTURIST!

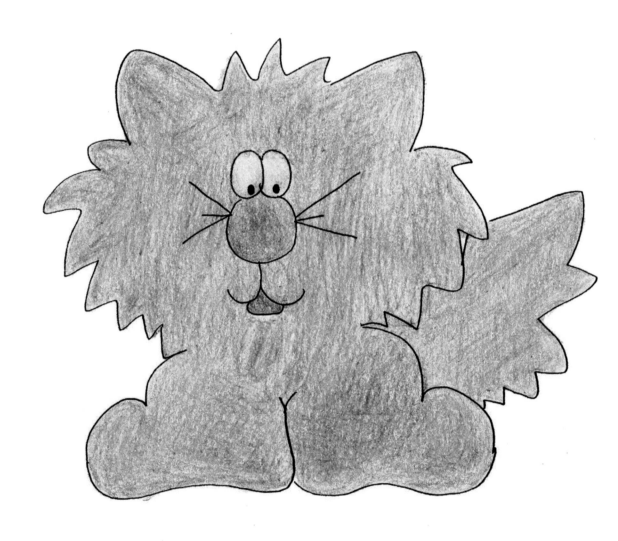

CAN I GO WITH YOU ON YOUR NEXT VISIT TO
THE ACUPUNCTURIST?

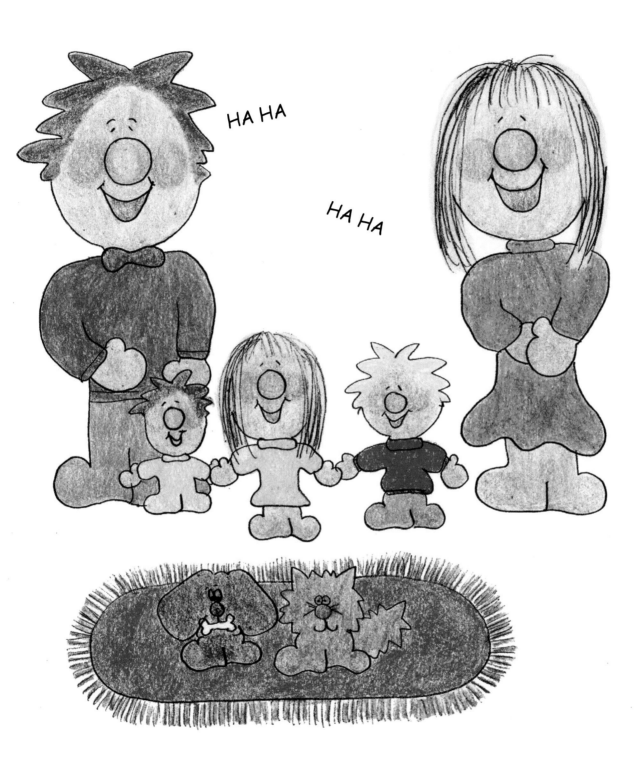

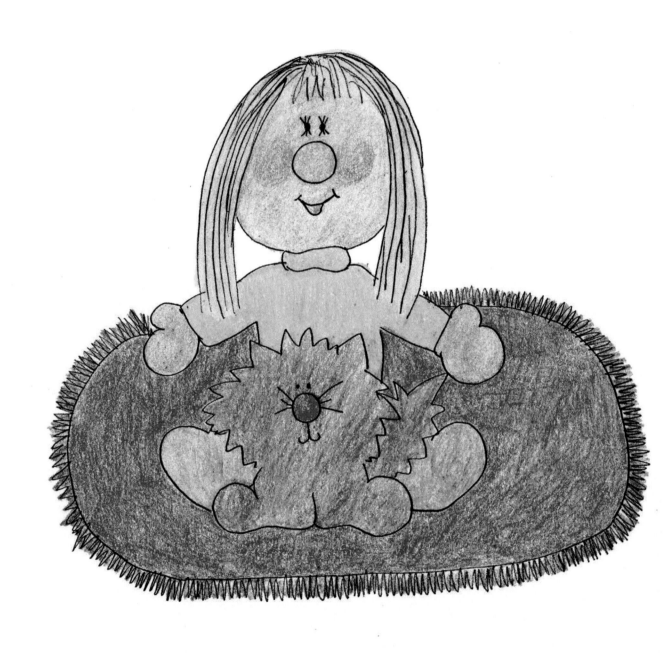

YOU SILLY CAT! YOU WOULD VISIT AN ANIMAL DOCTOR.

Printed in the United States
by Baker & Taylor Publisher Services

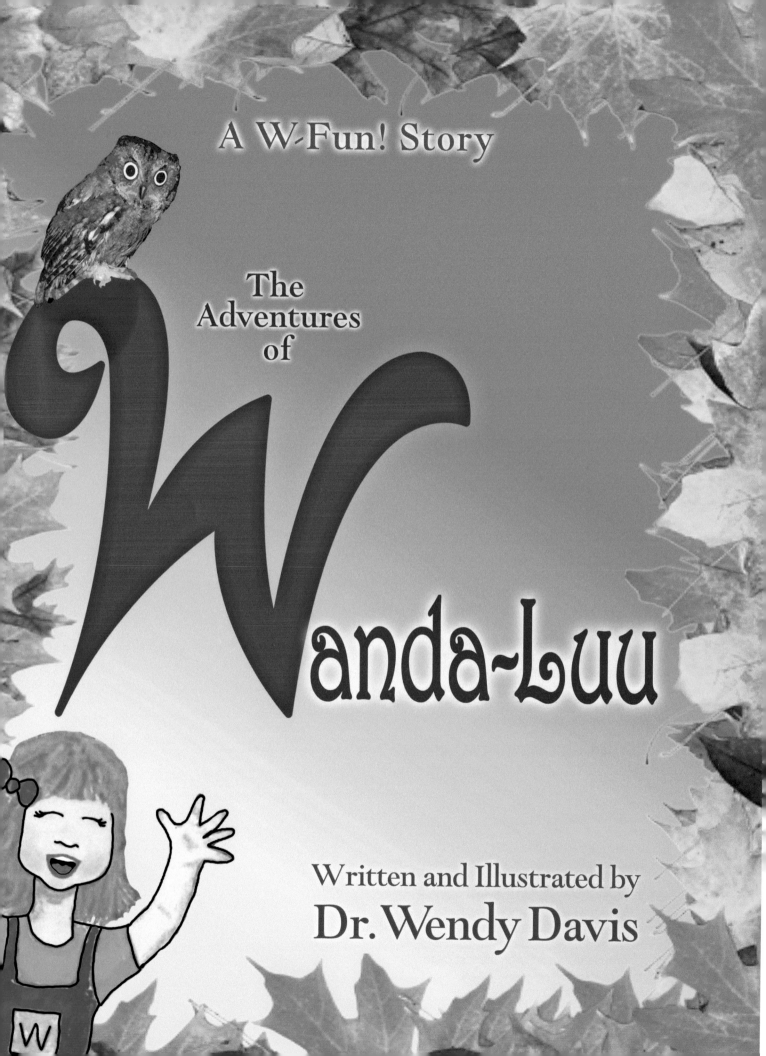

To order additional copies of this book, contact:
Xlibris
844-714-8691
www.Xlibris.com
Orders@Xlibris.com

Book Designer: Rick Contreras
Art Director: Mike Nardone

ISBN: Softcover   978-1-4010-6208-8

Library of Congress Control Number: 2002096169

Print information available on the last page

Rev. date: 03/19/2021